A
LITTLE BOOK
ON THE
HUMAN SHADOW

A LITTLE BOOK
ON THE
HUMAN SHADOW

ROBERT BLY

Edited by
William Booth

1817

Harper & Row, Publishers, San Francisco

Cambridge, Hagerstown, New York, Philadelphia, Washington
London, Mexico City, São Paulo, Singapore, Sydney

Grateful acknowledgement is given for permission to reprint: "Snowbanks North of the House" © 1975 by World Poetry, Inc. and "For My Son, Noah, Ten Years Old," copyright © 1979 by Holy Cow! Press. From the book: *The Man in the Black Coat Turns* by Robert Bly. Reprinted by permission of Doubleday, a division of Bantam, Doubleday, Dell Publishing Group, Inc. "Where We Must Look for Help," "Snowfall in the Afternoon," "Poem in Three Parts," and "Unrest," from *Silence in the Snowy Fields* (Middletown, Conn.: Wesleyan University Press, 1962; London: Cape, 1967). Copyright © 1960, 1961, 1962 by Robert Bly, reprinted with his permission. "The Moon" first appeared in *Kayak* 1, Autumn, 1964. Copyright © 1968 by Robert Bly, reprinted with his permission. "Sitting in his dentist's waiting room" is copyright © 1988 by Robert Bly, used by his permission. The essay "Wallace Stevens and Dr. Jekyll" first appeared in *American Poets in 1976*, edited by William Heyen (Bobs-Merrill, 1976). "The Busy Man Speaks," "Counting Small-Boned Bodies," "Hatred of Men With Black Hair," from *The Light Around the Body* (New York: Harper & Row, Publishers, Inc. 1967: London: Rapp & Whiting, 1968). Copyright © 1967 by Robert Bly. Used by permission of Harper & Row, Publishers, Inc. "Pilgrim Fish Heads" from *Sleepers Joining Hands* (New York, Harper & Row, Publishers, Inc., 1975). Copyright © 1975 by Robert Bly. Used by permission of Harper & Row, Publishers, Inc. Parts 1–4 of this book first appeared in chapbook form in issue 19 of *Raccoon*, published by Raccoon Books, Inc.

Library of Congress Cataloging-in-Publication Data

Bly, Robert.
    A little book on the human shadow.

    I. Booth, William   II. Title.
PS3552.L9L537   1988   814'.54   87-45687
ISBN 0-06-254847-6

88 89 90 91 92 MPC 10 9 8 7 6 5 4 3

Contents

Foreword

Whaat Robert Bly's poetry readings say in effect is, "You must change your life." To hear serious poems and resist all change is worse than a waste of time; it is dangerous. We can remember the warning from Jacob Boehme: "Boehme has a note before one of his books in which he asks the reader not to go further and read the book unless he is willing to make practical changes as a result of the reading. Otherwise, Boehme says, the book will be bad for him. . . ."

The reference to Boehme's unsettling words appears in Robert Bly's brilliant essay on the poetry of Wallace Stevens (part five of this book). In "Wallace Stevens and Dr. Jekyll," Bly praises Steven's extraordinary sensory intelligence, but says that his failure to "change his life" was disastrous to his later poetry. "Shadow" is the key word in Bly's assessment of the poet: Stevens brought the shadow into his poetry but shut it out of his everyday life. Bly's tough judgment of Steven's work after he failed to "live the shadow" is that "the late poems are as weak as is possible for a genius to write."

"Shadow" is one of Carl Jung's most useful terms for a part of the human psyche. Its advantage is that it conveys a visual image—we might call the shadow "the dark, unlit, and repressed side of the ego complex," the Jungian analyst Marie Louise von Franz says in *Shadow and Evil in Fairy Tales*. "But this is only partly true," she adds, lest we get caught in the negative connotation of the image. She tells of an occasion when Jung, impatient as

· 1 ·

always with Jungians, dismissed a nit-picking discussion of the concept by protesting, "This is all nonsense! The shadow is simply the whole unconscious." The definition Von Franz settles on is neutral and lucid: ". . . in the first stage of approach to the unconscious, the shadow is simply a 'mythological' name for all that within me of which I cannot directly know."

Robert Bly's intense interest in the concept of the human shadow goes back to early years when he lived alone in New York City. He has often spoken of this bleak period of his life, recalling an awareness of his own relationship to the shadow as one of the first things he understood clearly for himself. He knew that "if any help was going to arrive to lift me out of my misery, it would come from the dark side of my personality." The quotation is from the 1971 poetry reading where he first chose the shadow as a thematic image. He took up the theme in three subsequent readings, though the selection of poems changed and his accompanying commentary grew.

In the present collection of Bly's explorations of the shadow there is more poetry and storytelling than doctrinaire psychological discourse. He moves from image to image, and from image to anecdote and fairy tale. The shadow is "the long bag we drag behind us," heavy with the parts of ourselves our parents or community didn't approve of. The shadow is also imagined as a thin gray film rolled up in a can, out of sight, but ready to transfix us with lifelike images thrown onto a giant screen or played on a wife or husband's face. The long-repressed shadow of Dr. Jekyll rises up in the shape of Mr. Hyde, deformed, an ape-like figure glimpsed against an alley wall. Bly goes beyond such vivid evocation of the shadow's meaning in part three of this book ("Five Stages in Exiling, Hunting, and Retrieving the Shadow"), showing what one can do to change one's life, call up the energy lost in the shadow, bring back the witch and the giant.

Gathering the shadow readings into a book was a thought that came out of conversations I had with Roger Easson, who has done extensive bibliographical research into Bly's publications and recorded readings. Initially it seemed a simple enough matter to transcribe two or three readings, do some editing for the sake of sharper focus, and make the readings available in print.

When Bly saw the transcriptions that Easson and I had done, he was more distressed than we about what had been lost between the stage and the page—voice, music, gesture, interchange with the audience, all those nonverbal elements that convey meaning and feeling. Extensive revision followed. While the substance of the first three sections of this book is faithful to the original readings, Bly's revisions have brought them closer to the essay form.

The first part of this collection, "Problems in the Ark," is based on a studio reading recorded for the series "Contemporary American Poets Read Their Works," issued by Cassette Curriculum in 1971. Parts two and three are adapted from a reading given for a conference in San Francisco on "The Face of the Enemy," January 30, 1983. Part four is a conversation that Bly and I had about the shadow a year or so later. Part five, where Bly lets go the reader's hand and moves swiftly ahead into the shadowy forest of Wallace Steven's poetry, first appeared in *American Poetry in 1976,* edited by William Heyen.

—William Booth

PART 1

Problems in the Ark

1

Problems in the Ark

We notice that when sunlight hits the body, the body turns bright, but it throws a shadow, which is dark. The brighter the light, the darker the shadow. Each of us has some part of our personality that is hidden from us. Parents, and teachers in general, urge us to develop the light side of the personality—move into well-lit subjects such as mathematics and geometry—and to become successful. The dark part then becomes starved. What do we do then? We send out a crow.

> The dove returns: it found no resting place;
> It was in flight all night above the shaken seas;
> Beneath dark eaves
> The dove shall magnify the tiger's bed;
> Give the dove peace.
> The split-tailed swallow leaves the sill at dawn;
> At dusk, blue swallows shall return.
> On the third day the crow shall fly,
> The crow, the crow, the spider-colored crow,
> The crow shall find new mud to walk upon.

The poem refers to the Noah story, though I drew the images from an earlier version composed by the Babylonians, in which three birds took part. The poem came two or three years after college, and it seems to say that if any help was going to arrive to lift me out of my misery, it would come from the dark side of my personality. I remember this as one of the first things I understood clearly for myself. I felt that it was true also in politics—that is, what we needed to help us in the nation was not someone like Adlai Stevenson, who was too much like a swallow, or Bertrand Russell, who had too much light in his personality. Even Eugene McCarthy later on, who had a little more of the dark side, seemed to me a swallow, unable to find mud. Birds have become a problem for the United States. All we elect to the Presidency are doves or swallows, or white crows like Nixon.

One afternoon, several years later, watching snow fall on some long grass, I felt the positive dark come in again.

I

The grass is half-covered with snow.
It was the sort of snowfall that starts in late afternoon,
And now the little houses of the grass are growing dark.

II

If I reached my hands down, near the earth,
I could take handfuls of darkness!
A darkness was always there, which we never noticed.

III

As the snow grows heavier, the cornstalks fade farther away,
And the barn moves nearer to the house.
The barn moves all alone in the growing storm.

IV

The barn is full of corn, and moving toward us now,
Like a hulk blown toward us in a storm at sea;
All the sailors on deck have been blind for many years.

Sometimes the first snow comes while the grass is still green, and if the grass is long, bends it over, making little houses underneath. The barn at our farm that year was empty of animals, but full of corn, sealed in a government program, and though the corn belonged to my father, it was a sort of treasure. The image "handfuls of darkness" does not by itself make this a shadow poem. The poem approaches the shadow at the end as the writer gets more darkness than he bargained for.

The ancient Chinese culture emphasizes the Yin-Yang symbol, which shows us the white part of the personality and the black part of the personality united inside a circle. I wrote this poem one spring day.

I

Oh, on an early morning I think I shall live forever!
I am wrapped in my joyful flesh,
As the grass is wrapped in its clouds of green.

II

Rising from a bed where I dreamt
Of long rides past castles and hot coals,
The sun lies happily on my knees:
I have suffered and survived the night,
Bathed in dark water, like any blade of grass.

III

The strong leaves of the box-elder tree,
Plunging in the wind, call us to disappear
Into the wilds of the universe,
Where we shall sit at the foot of a plant,
And live forever, like the dust.

One could speculate that because ancient Chinese poets, Buddhist and non-Buddhist, tried to reconcile the dark side and the light side, they preserved more feeling for plants and animals than we have preserved. Plants are asleep, and so they live always in the dark side, though their leaves reach out for the light. So we could say that each weed in our back yard unites dark and light as the rose window of Chartres does, and sitting by them is much cheaper than flying over to France.

The Busy Man Speaks

Not to the mother of solitude will I give myself
Away, not to the mother of love, nor to the mother of
   conversation,
Nor to the mother of art, nor the mother
Of tears, nor the mother of the ocean;
Not to the mother of sorrow, nor the mother
Of the downcast face, nor the mother of the suffering of death;
Not to the mother of the night full of crickets,
Nor the mother of the open fields, nor the mother of Christ.

But I will give myself to the father of righteousness, the father
of cheerfulness, who is also the father of rocks,
Who is also the father of perfect gestures;
From the Chase National Bank
An arm of flame has come, and I am drawn
to the desert, to the parched places, to the landscape of zeros;
And I shall give myself away to the father of righteousness,
The stones of cheerfulness, the steel of money, the father of
   rocks.

Our culture teaches us from early infancy to split and polarize dark and light, which I call here "mother" and "father." So some people admire the right-thinking, well-lit side of the personality, and that group one can associate with the father, if one wants to; and some admire the left-thinking, poorly-lit side, and that group one can associate with the mother, if one wants to, and mythologically with the Great Mother. Most artists, poets, and musicians belong to the second group and love intuition, music, the feminine, owls, and the ocean. The right-thinking group loves action, commerce, and Empire. You see how my mind is split, so that my description of the world encourages polarization. I longed for a poem in which this split would be clear. The speaker in my poem would have to be an extraordinarily conscious father-type, I expect, but the poem reminds us that there are people who make a decision to cut themselves off from the darkness. I'll read a poem about early Pilgrim villages in Massachusetts.

It is a Pilgrim village; heavy rain is falling.
Fish heads lie smiling at the corners of houses.
Inside, words like "Samson" hang from the rafters.
Outdoors the chickens squawk in woody hovels,
yet the chickens are walking on Calvinist ground.
The women move through the dark kitchen, their heavy
skirts bear them down like drowning men.
Upstairs beds are like thunderclouds on the bare floor,
leaving the covers always moist by the rough wood.
And the eggs! Strange, white, perfect eggs!
Eggs that even the rain could not move,
white, painless, with tails even in nightmares.
And the Indian, damp, musky, asking for a bed.
The Mattapoiset is in league with rotting wood,
he has made a conspiracy with the salamander,
he has made treaties with the cold heads of fishes.
The Indian goes on living in the rain-soaked stumps.
This is our enemy, this is the outcast,
the one from whom we must protect our nation,
the one whose dark hair hides us from the sun.

I think one could say that most Puritans did not distinguish darkness from Satan. They feared swarthy Indians, probably were suspicious of dark-feathered turkeys, and walked uneasily in the pitchy pine woods of Massachusetts. For women they advised stockings, hoods, obedience, and silence. Hatred of the Yin side of the circle begins as a small thread in the first American cloth. Hatred of Yin at the start gave New England a fierce energy; but three hundred years later, the same hatred drains people and leads to some sort of spiritual death.

Sitting in his dentist's waiting room
it seems to him his life has run out.
One day, when he is forty-five,
the threshing floor sinks from sight,
and he can speak no longer.
He sits in a chair beneath great trees.
His wife gathers faggots in the woods.

Some American men enter a witchlike mythical space after forty-five. Men in many primitive cultures by contrast remain spiritually alive until they are seventy or eighty years old, as Buddhist priests often do, but with us, some speechlessness takes over. That dead space inside older American men is connected somehow to the old men's pursuit of the Vietnam War, and the way they pursued it, which was a numb, dead way. A perfect example of that numbness and deadness was the counting of the bodies.

Let's count the bodies over again.

If we could only make the bodies smaller,
The size of skulls,
We could make a whole plain white with skulls in the
  moonlight!

If we could only make the bodies smaller,
Maybe we could get
A whole year's kill in front of us on a desk!

If we could only make the bodies smaller,
We could fit
A body into a finger ring—for a keepsake—forever.

If the American drama begins with the Puritans killing turkeys, then Kissinger's and Nixon's bombing of Cambodia takes place in the third act. The South Asians, representing a civilization more reconciled to the moist dark than ours, merged with ghostly Cherokees or Crows far down in our psyche. During the

Vietnam War we listened every day to brutalizing body tallies, and I felt, and still feel, that the dreamlike quality of the war represented a repetition of some earlier massacres, as Sisyphus cannot stop pushing the stone up the hill in the underworld.

I hear voices praising Tshombe, and the Portuguese
In Angola, these are the men who skinned Little Crow!
We are all their sons, skulking
In back rooms, selling nails with trembling hands!

We distrust every person on earth with black hair;
We send teams to overthrow Chief Joseph's government;
We train natives to kill Presidents with blowdarts;
We have men loosening the nails on Noah's ark.

The State Department men float in the heavy jellies near
the bottom
Like exhausted crustaceans, like squids who are confused,
Sending out beams of black light to the open sea.
Each fights his fraternal feeling for the great landlords.

We have violet rays that light up the jungles at night,
showing us
The friendly populations; we are teaching the children of
ritual, the forest children,
To overcome their longing for life, and we send
Sparks of black light that fit the holes in the generals' eyes.

Underneath all the cement of the Pentagon
There is a drop of Indian blood preserved in snow:
Preserved from a trail of blood that once led away
From the stockade, over the snow, the trail now lost.

The Sioux leader Little Crow mentioned in the second line led a brief rebellion in Minnesota during the Civil War, which was put down. Several years later a white farmer shot Little Crow when he happened on him one day picking blackberries. When he brought Little Crow's body into town, a former soldier recognized him by the skunk fur bands on his wrists. The farmers beheaded Little Crow and then skinned him, and the Minnesota Historical Society had the skin for a while. The detail is curiously like the ear-cutting that went on in Vietnam.

So a decision taken privately, as a part of one's inner life, to fight the dark side of oneself—and this fight the Protestants particularly recommended—can cause "the conscious" and "the unconscious" to take up adversary positions; and the adversary positions can quickly spread to foreign policy, and influence decisions. The crow doesn't arrive: we divide animals in the Ark into good and bad, but the crow doesn't arrive. We make all the male porcupines and sloths sit on the right side of the room, and the female porcupines and sloths on the left side of the room, but the crow doesn't arrive. The two halves of Yin and Yang do not join. We forbid the herons to dance, and we force the mice in their crowded quarters to bring all mice infants to full term, but the crow still doesn't arrive. What do we do then, to encourage the crow to arrive? That is the subject of this little book. The division insisted on here of dark and light is very stark, but that's how we'll begin.

PART 2

The Long Bag We Drag Behind Us

2

The Long Bag We Drag Behind Us

It's an old Gnostic tradition that we don't invent things, we just remember. The Europeans I know of who remember the dark side best are Robert Louis Stevenson, Joseph Conrad, and Carl Jung. I'll call up a few of their ideas and add a few thoughts of my own.

Let's talk about the personal shadow first. When we were one or two years old we had what we might visualize as a 360-degree personality. Energy radiated out from all parts of our body and all parts of our psyche. A child running is a living globe of energy. We had a ball of energy, all right; but one day we noticed that our parents didn't like certain parts of that ball. They said things like: "Can't you be still?" Or "It isn't nice to try and kill your brother." Behind us we have an invisible bag, and the part of us our parents don't like, we, to keep our parents' love, put in the bag. By the time we go to school our bag is quite large. Then our teachers have their say: "Good children don't get angry over such little things." So we take our anger and put it in the bag. By the time my brother and I were twelve in Madison, Minnesota we were known as "the nice Bly boys." Our bags were already a mile long.

Then we do a lot of bag-stuffing in high school. This time it's no longer the evil grownups that pressure us, but people our own age. So the student's paranoia about grownups can be misplaced. I lied all through high school automatically to try to be more like the basketball players. Any part of myself that was a little slow went into the bag. My sons are going through the process now; I watched my daughters, who were older, experience it. I noticed with dismay how much they put into the bag, but there was nothing their mother or I could do about it. Often my daughters seemed to make their decision on the issue of fashion and collective ideas of beauty, and they suffered as much damage from other girls as they did from men.

So I maintain that out of a round globe of energy the twenty-year-old ends up with a slice. We'll imagine a man who has a thin slice left—the rest is in the bag—and we'll imagine that he meets a woman; let's say they are both twenty-four. She has a thin, elegant slice left. They join each other in a ceremony, and this union of two slices is called marriage. Even together the two do not make up one person! Marriage when the bag is large entails loneliness during the honeymoon for that very reason. Of course we all lie about it. "How is your honeymoon?" "Wonderful, how's yours?"

Different cultures fill the bag with different contents. In Christian culture sexuality usually goes into the bag. With it goes much spontaneity. Marie Louise von Franz warns us, on the other hand, not to sentimentalize primitive cultures by assuming that they have no bag at all. She says in effect that they have a different but sometimes even larger bag. They may put individuality into the bag, or inventiveness. What anthropologists know as "participation mystique," or "a mysterious communal mind," sounds lovely, but it can mean that tribal members all know exactly the same thing and no one knows anything else. It's possible that bags for all human beings are about the same size.

We spend our life until we're twenty deciding what parts of ourself to put into the bag, and we spend the rest of our lives trying to get them out again. Sometimes retrieving them feels impossible, as if the bag were sealed. Suppose the bag remains sealed—what happens then? A great nineteenth-century story has an idea about that. One night Robert Louis Stevenson woke up and told his wife a bit of a dream he'd just had. She urged him to write it down; he did, and it became "Dr. Jekyll and Mr. Hyde." The nice side of the personality becomes, in our idealistic culture, nicer and nicer. The Western man may be a liberal doctor, for example, always thinking about the good of others. Morally and ethically he is wonderful. But the substance in the bag takes on a personality of its own; it can't be ignored. The story says that the substance locked in the bag appears one day *somewhere else* in the city. The substance in the bag feels angry, and when you see it it is shaped like an ape, and moves like an ape.

The story says then that when we put a part of ourselves in the bag it regresses. It de-evolves toward barbarism. Suppose a young man seals a bag at twenty and then waits fifteen or twenty years before he opens it again. What will he find? Sadly, the sexuality, the wildness, the impulsiveness, the anger, the freedom he put in have all regressed; they are not only primitive in mood, they are hostile to the person who opens the bag. The man who opens his bag at forty-five or the woman who opens her bag rightly feels fear. She glances up and sees the shadow of an ape passing along the alley wall; anyone seeing that would be frightened.

I think we could say that most males in our culture put their feminine side or interior woman into the bag. When they begin, perhaps around thirty-five or forty, trying to get in touch with their feminine side again, she may be by then truly hostile to them. The same man may experience in the meantime much hostility from women in the outer world. The rule seems to be: the outside has to be like the inside. That's the way it is on this globe. If a woman, wanting to be approved for her femininity, has put her masculine side or her internal male into the bag, she may find that twenty years later he will be hostile to her. Moreover he may be unfeeling and brutal in his criticism. She's in a spot. Finding a hostile man to live with would give her someone to blame, and take away the pressure, but that wouldn't help the problem of the closed bag. In the meantime, she is liable to sense a double rejection, from the male inside and the male outside. There's a lot of grief in this whole thing.

Every part of our personality that we do not love will become hostile to us. We could add that it may move to a distant place and begin a revolt against us as well. A lot of the trouble Shakespeare's kings experience blossoms in that sentence. Hotspur "in Wales" rebels against the King. Shakespeare's poetry is marvelously sensitive to the danger of these inner revolts. Always the king at the center is endangered.

When I visited Bali a few years ago, it became clear that their ancient Hindu culture works through mythology to bring shadow elements up into daily view. The temples put on plays virtually every day from the *Ramayana*. I saw some terrifying plays performed as a part of religious life, in a day by day way. Almost every Balinese house has standing outside it a fierce, toothy, aggressive, hostile figure carved in stone. This being doesn't plan to do good. I visited a mask maker, and noticed his nine- or ten-year-old son sitting outside the house, making with his chisel a hostile, angry figure. The person does not aim to act out the aggressive energies as we do in football or the Spanish in bullfighting, but each person aims to bring them upward into art: that is the ideal. The Balinese can be violent and brutal in war, but in daily life they seem much less violent than we are. What can this mean? Southerners in the United States put figures of helpful little black men on the lawn, cast in iron, and we in the North do the same with serene deer. We ask for roses in the wallpaper, Renoir above the sofa, and John Denver on the stereo. Then the aggression escapes from the bag and attacks everyone.

We'll have to let this contrast between Balinese and American cultures lie there and go on. I want to talk about the connection between shadow energies and the moving picture projector. Let's suppose that we have miniaturized certain parts of ourselves, flattened them out, and put them inside a can, where it will be dark. Then one night—always at night—the shapes reappear, huge, and we can't take our eyes away from them. We drive at night in the country and see a man and woman on an enormous outdoor movie screen; we shut off the car and watch. Certain figures who have been rolled up inside a can, doubly invisible by being partially "developed" and by being kept always in the dark, exist during the day only as pale images on a thin gray strip of film. When a certain light is ignited in the back of our heads, ghostly pictures appear on a wall in front of us. They light cigarettes; they threaten others with guns. Our psyches then are natural projection machines: images that we stored in a can we can bring out while still rolled up, and run them for others, or on others. A man's anger, rolled up inside the can for twenty years, he may see one night on his wife's face. A wife might see a hero every night on her husband's face and then one night see a tyrant. Nora in *A Doll's House* saw the two images in turn.

The other day I found some of my old diaries, and I picked out one at random, from 1956. I had been struggling that year to write a poem describing the nature of advertising men. I remember that, and I recall that at that time the story of Midas was important in my mood. Everything that Midas touched turned to gold. I declared in my poem that every living thing an advertising man touches turns into some form of money, and that's why ad men have such starved souls. I kept in mind the ad men I'd known and was having a good time attacking them from my concealed position. As I read the old passages I felt a shock seeing the movie I was running. Between the time I wrote them and now I'd discovered that I had known for years how to eat in such a way as to keep me from taking in any kind of nourishment. Whatever food a friend offered me, or a woman, or a child, turned into metal on the way to my mouth. Is the image clear? No one can eat or drink metal. So Midas was a good image for me. But the film showing my interior Midas was rolled up in the can. Advertising men, evil and foolish, tended to appear at night on a large screen, and I was naturally fascinated. A year or two later I composed a book called *Poems for the*

Ascension of J. P. Morgan, in which each poem I had written about business alternated with a culpable advertisement reproduced from magazines or newspapers. It is a lively book in its way. No one would publish it, but that was all right. It was mostly projection anyway. I'm going to read you a poem I wrote around that time. It's called "Unrest."

A strange unrest hovers over the nation:
This is the last dance, the wild tossing of Morgan's seas,
The division of spoils. A lassitude
Enters into the diamonds of the body.
In high school the explosion begins, the child is partly killed;
When the fight is over, and the land and the sea ruined,
Two shapes inside us rise, and move away.

But the baboon whistles on the shores of death—
Climbing and falling, tossing nuts and stones,
He gambols by the tree
Whose branches hold the expanses of cold,
The planets whirling and the black sun,
The cries of insects, and the tiny slaves
In the prisons of bark.
Charlemagne, we are approaching your islands!

(I got a little rhetorical in that stanza.)

We are returning now to the snowy trees,
And the depth of the darkness buried in snow, through
   which you rode all night
With stiff hands; now the darkness is falling
In which we sleep and awake—a darkness in which
Thieves shudder, and the insane have a hunger for snow,
In which bankers dream of being buried by black stones,
And businessmen fall on their knees in the dungeons of sleep.

About five years ago I began to be suspicious of this poem. Why are bankers and businessmen being singled out? If I had to rephrase "banker" what would I say? "Someone who plans very well." I plan very well. How would I rephrase "businessman"? "Someone with a stiff face." I looked in the mirror then. I'll read you the way the passage goes now, after I've rewritten it:

. . . a darkness in which
Thieves shudder, and the insane have a hunger for snow,
In which good planners dream of being buried by black stones,
And men with stiff faces like me fall on their knees in the
    dungeons of sleep.

Now when I go to a party I feel different from the way than I used to when I meet a businessman. I say to a man, "What do you do?" He says, "I'm a stockbroker." And he says it in a faintly apologetic way. I say to myself, "Look at this: something of me that was deep inside me is standing right next to me." I have a funny longing to hug him. Not all of them, of course.

But projection is a wonderful thing too. Marie Louise von Franz remarked somewhere, "Why do we always assume projection is bad? 'You are projecting' becomes among Jungians an accusation. Sometimes projection is helpful and the right thing." Her remark is very wise. I know that I was starving myself to death, but the knowledge couldn't move directly from the bag to the conscious mind. It has to go out onto the world first. "How wicked advertising men are," I said to myself. Marie Louise von Franz reminds us that if we didn't project, we might never connect with the world at all. Women sometimes complain that a man often takes his ideal feminine side and projects it onto a woman. But if he didn't, how could he get out of his mother's house or his bachelor room? The issue is not so much that we do project but how long we keep the projections out there. Projection without personal contact is dangerous. Thousands, even millions of American men projected their internal feminine onto Marilyn Monroe. If a million men do that, and leave it there, it's likely she will die. She died. Projections without personal contact can damage the person receiving them.

We have to say also that Marilyn Monroe called for these projections as a part of her power longing, and her disturbance must have gone back to victimization in childhood. But the process of projection and recall, done so delicately in tribal culture, face to face, goes out of whack when the mass media arrives. In the economy of the psyche her death was inevitable and even right. No single human being can carry so many projections—that is, so much unconsciousness—and survive. So it's infinitely important that each person bring back his or her own.

But why would we give away, or put into the bag, so much of ourselves? Why would we do it so young? And if we have put away so many of our angers, spontaneities, hungers, enthusiasms, our rowdy and unattractive parts, then how can we live? What holds us together? Alice Miller spoke to this point in her book *Prisoners of Childhood*, which in paperback form is called *The Drama of the Gifted Child*.

The drama is this. We came as infants "trailing clouds of glory," arriving from the farthest reaches of the universe, bringing with us appetites well preserved from our mammal inheritance, spontaneities wonderfully preserved from our 150,000 years of tree life, angers well preserved from our 5,000 years of tribal life—in short, with our 360-degree radiance—and we offered this gift to our parents. They didn't want it. They wanted a nice girl or a nice boy. That's the first act of the drama. It doesn't mean our parents were wicked; they needed us for something. My mother, as a second generation immigrant, needed my brother and me to help the family look more classy. We do the same thing to our children; it's a part of life on this planet. Our parents rejected who we were before we could talk, so the pain of the rejection is probably stored in some pre-verbal place.

When I read her book I fell into depression for three weeks. With so much gone, what can we do? We can construct a personality more acceptable to our parents. Alice Miller agrees that we have betrayed ourselves, but she says, "Don't blame yourself for that. There's nothing else you could have done." Children in ancient times who opposed their parents probably were set out to die. We did, as children, the only sensible thing under the circumstances. The proper attitude toward that, she says, is mourning.

Let's talk now about the different sorts of bags. When we have put a lot in our private bag, we often have as a result little energy. The bigger the bag, the less the energy. Some people have by nature more energy than others, but we all have more than we can possibly use. Where did it go? If we put our sexuality into the bag as a child, obviously we lose with it a lot of energy. When a woman puts her masculinity into the bag, or rolls it up and puts it into the can, she loses energy with it. So we can think of our personal bag as containing energy now unavailable to us. If we identify ourselves as uncreative, it means we took our creativity and put it into the bag. What do you mean, "I am not creative"? "Let experts do it"—isn't that what such a person is saying? That's damn well what such people are saying. The audience wants a poet, a hired gun, to come in from out of town. Everybody in this audience should be writing their own poems.

We have talked of our personal bag, but each town or community also seems to have a bag. I lived for years near a small Minnesota farm town. Everyone in the town was expected to have the same objects in the bag; a small Greek town clearly would have different objects in the bag. It's as if the town, by collective psychic decision, puts certain energies in the bag, and tries to prevent anyone from getting them out. Towns interfere with our private process in this matter, so it's more dangerous to live in them than in nature. On the other hand, certain ferocious hatreds that one feels in a small town help one sometimes to see where the projections have gone. And the Jungian community, like the town, has its bag, and usually recommends that Jungians keep their vulgarity and love of money in the bag; and the

Freudian community usually demands that Freudians keep their religious life in the bag.

There is also a national bag, and ours is quite long. Russia and China have noticeable faults, but if an American citizen is curious to know what is in our national bag at the moment, he can listen closely when a State Department official criticizes Russia. As Reagan says, we are noble; other nations have empires. Other nations endure stagnated leadership, treat minorities brutally, brainwash their youth, and break treaties. A Russian can find out about his bag by reading a *Pravda* article on the United States. We're dealing with a network of shadows, a pattern of shadows projected by both sides, all meeting somewhere out in the air. I'm not saying anything new with this metaphor, but I do want to make the distinction clear between the personal shadow, the town shadow, and the national shadow.

I have used three metaphors here: the bag, the film can, and projection. Since the can or bag is closed and its images remain in the dark, we can only see the contents of our own bag by throwing them innocently, as we say, out into the world. Spiders then become evil, snakes cunning, goats oversexed; men become linear, women become weak, the Russians become unprincipled, and Chinese all look alike. Yet it is precisely through this expensive, damaging, wasteful, inaccurate form of mud-slinging that we eventually come in touch with the mud that the crow found on the bottom of his feet.

PART 3

Five Stages in Exiling, Hunting, and Retrieving the Shadow

3

Five Stages in Exiling, Hunting, and Retrieving the Shadow

When one "projects," one is really giving away an energy or power that rightfully belongs to one's own treasury. A man may give his "feeling side" or "relationship mode" away to his wife. Then he is rid of it, and when a feeling problem with the children comes up, he naturally lets her handle the problem.

What other qualities or powers does a man project onto a woman? He may project animal sexuality onto her, in which case she may feel wicked and overly animal; he may project spirituality onto her, in which case she will feel unduly elevated; he may give her his power of weakness, or his insanity. Some men project their competence in the world onto a woman. And many men give their witch to a woman, or to several women.

As for a woman, she may project her interior hero onto her husband, in which case he will feel overly noble and responsible; she may project her Saturn onto a man, so that she may remain playful and whimsical, but he will grow more and more rigid; she may give him her internal tyrant, or her spirituality; she may project her hatred of relationship onto him, so that he feels excessively cold and unrelated; and many women give their giant to a man, or to several men.

We all know a lot about giving away our power, but in this talk we will discuss ways of getting those given-away powers back. We will follow the adventures of a man who has given his witch away, and a woman who has given her giant or tyrant away. But the process of giving and reabsorbing projected substances is similar for all the qualities we have scattered out into the world, whether projected on people of the other sex, on children, on parents, on teachers, on races, or on nations.

I'll suggest, then, five stages, beginning with the stage in which the psyche has sent the unwelcome power out and it is successfully projected. When the uncomfortable talent is well exiled, all that is left inside is a thin, gray, wispy substance, hardly noticeable in daylight.

The male child begins projecting his interior witch early, perhaps at two or three months, the mother being a good hook. Some observers believe that the baby, when he or she experiences for the first time the mother's refusal of the breast, or some other setback, sees, his perceptions powered by enormous rage, fangs actually come out of her mouth, and skulls appear around her neck. Children feel grateful when a grownup reads witch stories to them because it proves to them that they are not insane. The child, male or female, lives with this secret, that the mother whom everyone declares to be supportive and caring has a witch face at times, and the child knows he is too small to do anything about it.

Some men let their mother carry their witch for the rest of their lives, but most men, when they marry, transfer their witch, or most of it, over to their new bride. While the bride and groom stand in front of the minister exchanging rings, another important exchange takes place in the basement. During a separate meeting, the mother passes over the son's witch, which she has been carrying, to the bride. An hour after the ceremony the witch is firmly in place inside the bride, though it will take a while for it to show up, because neither the bride, nor the mother, nor the groom knows about this second ceremony. But after a few arguments, a few obstinacies, and a few money fights, it occurs to the groom one day that there is something witch-like in his bride that he hadn't noticed before. It sometimes occurs to her too that something bizarre has happened. During an argument she feels herself more greedy, or more witchy. One woman said to me, "Robert, before I was married I was quite a nice person. But now I've been married for three years, and you know, I'm getting bitchier and bitchier. How can this be?" I said, "Well, you've been eating for two." The husband meanwhile gets sweeter and sweeter, and this enrages his wife still more, and tends to bring out more of her witch side. She is now carrying witchiness—that is, impulsive irritability, abrupt greediness, unfairness, unexplainable hostility, an underground current of rage—for both of them. He feels quite calm, and looks with wonder and pity on her behavior.

During the marriage service a similar exchange takes place between the groom and the bride's father. Perhaps their spirits meet in the garage—their actual bodies being in church—and the bride's father passes over to the groom as much as he can find of the giant or the tyrant that he has been carrying for his daughter. The bride's father leaves the church door lighter, the groom heavier. The groom receives from the father many other transferred projections as well: he may have to carry her spiritual guide, and perhaps her interior bluebeard, some brutal side of the feminine. Besides his childhood witch, the bride receives from the mother of the groom his helplessness, his deviousness, perhaps his Kali-like rage. The bride goes home from the wedding considerably heavier.

We'll call the first stage of projection then the state of mind in which shadow material, well handled by trained conspirators, comes to rest outside the owner's psyche, and seems likely to remain out there somewhere. The bride and groom may remain in this first stage for years. Some things, like the wedding silver, last a long time.

But sooner or later one of the projections starts to rattle, in the lovely word Marie Louise von Franz uses. Something doesn't quite fit any more, and we hear a rattle. We'll call this rattling the second stage. The man's wife acts witchy at times and not at other times, and no matter how much the husband squints at her through half closed eyes, she definitely is acting generously and not witchily. That is confusing for the man. He may begin, unconsciously of course, coming home late for dinner without telling her, or forgetting birthdays and anniversaries. Hopefully she'll take those rudenesses personally, and the mask will fit again.

It is threatening when the projection starts to rattle. Let's suppose a woman has put a giant's mask firmly on her husband's face, and feels it as a painful relief—at least she gets it out of her psyche. But what if her husband fails one day to be a negative patriarch? What to do then? Trouble. She might, unconsciously of course, overdraw her checking account, lose bills, dent the fender, feel victimized, act like a little girl. That may turn him into a tyrant again. Or she may go to a feminist meeting to be revved up. Hopefully someone there will explain that even men's kindnesses are a subtle part of their oppression. When she gets home he has the patriarch mask on again.

Archibald Cox described participating in a discussion of Russian-American relations with right wing fundamentalists in Orange County: they seemed convinced that the Russians broke every treaty, and he guessed that they expected him, as a former CIA man, to support their belief. When he reported in detail about a number of treaties the Russians had followed meticulously, the Orange County people got very upset, more upset than if he had told them the Russians intended to invade next month.

Many young American men and women in the last twenty years have projected their spiritual guide onto an Asian guru; that projection lasts a while, and then starts to rattle. Perhaps a student hears that his or her guru is sleeping with young girls, or buying Rolls-Royces by the dozen. An ashram of disciples may live for years in the anguish of the second stage.

What is the second stage like in our projections onto our children? A sort of history of child-rearing in Germany in the nineteenth century came out recently called *For Your Own Good*, written by Alice Miller. She notes that around 1850 the bad word in such circles was "exuberance." Some child-rearing books spoke of exuberance as if it were negative and potentially evil. The books would say, "Now when your child gets to be two or two and a half years old, you'll notice a lot of exuberance appearing. This is your test as a parent. If you fail this test the child will end in prison or drug addiction." Not all child psychologists of the time thought in this way, but many did, and their thought affected the lives of millions of children. One way of curing exuberance, they said, was to keep the severity of punishments unrelated to the offense. If the child spills milk, don't speak to the child for three days. (Ashley Montague, as you know, maintains that aggressive instincts belong to the human genetic inheritance, but that violence is learned, and learned in the family.)

So nineteenth-century Germans considered exuberance to be a form of wickedness, and that was a wickedness that they had already put into their bag, along with weakness, the desire to cry, the longing to get excited. It seems, then, that what women and men project onto children is wicked weakness. We believe secretly that our weakness as children was wicked. We should have been stronger; our pliability was evil. Our weakness was wicked. Children were considered evil in Salem, Massachusetts. It's important to have these two concepts, weakness and wickedness, together. We believe that it was wicked weakness that we had.

What then? We get angry at our children, especially those of our own sex. My oldest children were daughters, and I didn't feel that too much anger went toward them. Every parent knows the situation—more anger flies out of us than is justified by anything the child has done. Do you know that situation? Perhaps the child fails to finish his chores, or breaks a glass, and the parent goes wild. And what can the child do?—feel fear. I've seen it in my children's eyes, and I felt horror at that.

So when we can consider our children weak, wickedly weak,

we have gotten rid of something else that's in our bag. What a relief it is to be strong! But when it occurs to me that my children are not actually wicked, then I've got a problem, because I've passed into the second stage, and the substance is threatening to come back. This is a dangerous moment. We can become violent when there is a threat that we may have to take it back.

I've described the second stage as the state of mind in which there is some rattling, some troublesome inconsistency. A man's wife is carrying his witch, but she doesn't look or act like a witch all the time; the woman's husband is carrying her negative patriarch, but he doesn't look or act like a patriarch all the time; and we know dozens of other examples. China may act honorably; a right-winger may be compassionate, a leftist disciplined. This is distressing. In this stage one begins to get nervous, and anything can happen. All traces of exuberance, life-force, inconsistency, spontaneity become threatening.

I'll call the third stage that state of mind in which the distressed person calls on the moral intelligence to repair the rattle. The idea is scary because we need the moral intelligence, yet here it becomes a tool for continued unconsciousness. People with moral intelligence are often very dangerous types, because the moment the mask is about to fall off, they step forward on request to put it back. Walt Whitman Rostow was, during the Vietnam War, an example of such a person, as were the Alsop brothers. Lyndon Johnson felt that the Asians were ignoble, and we were noble. When our saturation bombing from high altitudes, use of napalm on civilians, and policy of village massacre began to cast doubt on that, Johnson began to compare himself to Lincoln, and Rostow spoke of moral fiber, duties of the peace-giving nation, etc. In child abuse the rule is: every act of cruelty, conscious or unconscious, that our parents take, we interpret as an act of love. So the moral intelligence redefines gross human abuse as an act of love.

And the anti-war protesters fell into the third stage also. When it appeared that not all policemen were pigs, that Ho Chi

Minh wasn't precisely Albert Schweitzer, that Hubert Humphrey had some honor even if he remained Vice President, then the moral intelligence rose to replace all masks, reject Humphrey, and effectively elect Nixon. Many leftists kept shouting, "America is spelled with a 'k'!" The left has a long bag, and can call on awesome moral intelligence to keep the projection going, to the enormous damage of both sides. The mask is put back on, for the best reasons, "for your own good." It is easy to fall into the third stage. Many times I heard policemen called pigs and didn't say a thing at the time.

Let's turn now to what we project onto children. When a child exhibits some wicked weakness, and yet we notice that our anger is far in excess of any appropriate response, then what? I found that a voice inside me would say: "Never mind. You're here to give discipline to this child! If you don't he'll be lazy and irresponsible."

Similarly students in the ashram who have become upset over the guru's behavior will soon begin justifying it. They have recourse to the wonderful resources of the moral intelligence. They'll tell you that he is exhibiting "crazy wisdom," or that he is doing what he's doing to challenge the "Western ego."

Let's recapitulate the stages I've suggested briefly. To start with, the man's witch and the woman's giant are out there, and that feels fine. Many qualities are projected. Nora gave her hero to Torvald, and he gave his childishness to her. Then the machine started to wobble a little, and Nora found out that sometimes Torvald was a hero and sometimes he wasn't. Nora then planned with her moral intelligence a crisis for Torvald in which he would prove triumphantly to be a magnificent hero. It didn't work. So the desperate effort in the third stage to refit the hero mask, search the memory for witch dangers, fight with all women against negative patriarchs, achieves its aim only for a short time.

What is the fourth stage? Suppose that one day, exhausted, one gives up for a moment the struggle to make the mask hang onto the other person. At that moment the eyes break contact; we suddenly look into ourselves and see our own diminishment. We recognize how diminished we have been for years. I would call the fourth stage the state of mind in which we feel the sensation of diminishment. If a boy has given his witch to his mother, and then, when older, has given it to his wife or lover, one day, perhaps at the age of thirty-five or forty, he will feel soft and diminished, precisely because his witch is out there. We can say that the witch corresponds to a force in us that wants to block our growth, yet we must say that the witch presents a very positive force also. Her value lies in the fact that she knows what she wants. "I want you to separate these seeds by sunset, and I'm going to eat you up if you don't." The witch doesn't say, "Well, let's just check the *I Ching* to see if you should separate these seeds." I've noticed recently that more and more agreeable men or "soft males" are turning up in the United States. I respect these men, because they have often developed their feminine selves in brave and original ways. Many American men have moved to do that, in ways hardly guessed at by French men or German men. And yet the fault of the soft male lies in what we could call the absence of the witch. If you ask such a man what he wants to do, he may say, "Well, I don't know, what would you like to do?" "I'll do what the others do." "I'll ask my girl friend." When the soft male loses a relationship, it is usually broken by the woman. At Lama Commune a man told me that every serious relationship there broken off in the last three years was broken by the woman. The soft male often doesn't have enough of the witch left to say, "Enough!" When the witch reenters we could say a certain crispness enters into the man. A man then who has projected his witch out eventually feels diminished; and it's very important that he feel that pain deeply, hold to it, keep the pain of it. He may notice that what he is best at is empathy, listening to others' pain, going with the flow; and he may be capable only of that, but the power the witch has to want what she wants, he doesn't possess.

We all understand how a woman who has given her hero to a man will later feel diminished, but giving the negative patriarch to a man or men is no better. When one gives the negative, one gives the positive also. Women who have projected the patriarch usually practice consensus in daily life: the talking solution, no one in authority, the circle in which everyone speaks, imagining that the matriarchy functioned this way. Consensus politics often works well in dealing with persons in daily life, but it doesn't work inside. When a woman practices consensus among her interior beings, the interior critic or bluebeard may simply move in and dismember her. Consensus politics doesn't work well inside men either, for the same reason. So by insisting that patriarchal authority is the primary evil in the world, and priding herself on having no part of such authority, a woman may condemn herself to brutalization by strong forces inside her, just as the soft male, because of his absent witch, lacks the strength to end a relationship that has turned into slavery, let alone end a relationship with interior beings that involve slavery.

If we have given away thirty parts of our self, we will then eventually feel ourselves diminished in thirty different ways. Men and women usually take back their spiritual guide from a guru when they feel sufficiently diminished. That doesn't mean they were wrong to give it to him in the first place, but the idea suggests that each student should be as alert to his or her diminishment as to the initial elevation or empowerment.

Our friends play crucial roles in what we called the fourth stage. The sense of diminishment sets up strange situations. If we tell a friend of our feeling, it's important that the friend not try to cheer us up at that point. "I don't think you've really lost anything; you're just a drip by nature." If a woman retrieves her patriarch, or a man retrieves his witch, their respective friends may not like it. Our friends are used to us as we are.

And what about children? They may get used to being wickedly weak, or at least ambiguously weak, and so freeze us into a position of being ethically strong. When we feel diminished in relation to our children, it's usually because we have given our child to them, and they, with the cunning of the child, dominate us. J. B. Yeats, W. B. Yeats's father, wrote to his son after living two years in the United States, "You know discipline is essential in every family. In Europe the children discipline themselves so that the parents can have a good time; in America the parents discipline themselves so the children can have a good time." Many American parents don't feel their diminishment in the presence of their children as diminishment, but feel it as a new way of parenting.

It's clear how diminished Reagan feels by projecting madness, cunning, spy-genius, military superiority, and superhuman cleverness onto the Russians; and so we allow Russia, as we allow our children, to set the tone in the house, and determine our expenditures.

We don't live wholly at any moment in the fourth stage or the fifth stage or any stage; we are in all five stages simultaneously, as we send out or receive back various rejected qualities, projected substances, abandoned powers, each absent in different degrees, or retrievable with different schedules.

It's clear that the fifth stage in this long process amounts to the state of mind in which we retrieve the giant, retrieve the hero, retrieve the witch, retrieve the wicked child, retrieve our brutal national character; and the whole process of retrieval could be called eating the shadow.

Eating our shadow is a very slow process. It doesn't happen once, but hundreds of times. Churchill said, "I have had to eat many of my own words, and I found the diet very nourishing."

Puritanism by its insistence that the child is truly wicked prevented many seventeenth-century Americans from eating that part of their shadow, and some malnourishment is evident in their literature. The witch-burning craze, pushed along by ignorant monks who had forgottten how to think mythologically, caused immense suffering and injustice, and prevented the men administering it from eating their own witch, and the church is still undernourished there.

As a person grows older he or she becomes more wise about this stage. The mother feeds, after all, but the witch eats. So the witch has to be brought back, I think, for the person to eat a significant portion of his or her shadow. When the person begins to bring in rejected or projected authority, for example, and eat that, Saturn enters, and our passion deepens, and melancholy, always a mark of Saturn, and of retrieved shadow, brings its sorrow in, and its opening to the spirit. We sense limits, and limits begin to seem a part of us, a natural agency of life. This poem is called "Snowbanks North of the House."

Those great sweeps of snow that stop suddenly six feet from
    the house . . .
Thoughts that go so far.
The boy gets out of high school and reads no more books;
the son stops calling home.
The mother puts down her rolling pin and makes no more
    bread.
And the wife looks at her husband one night at a party and
    loves him no more.
The energy leaves the wine, and the minister falls leaving the
    church.
It will not come closer—
the one inside moves back, and the hands touch nothing,
    and are safe.
The father grieves for his son, and will not leave the room
    where the coffin stands.
He turns away from his wife, and she sleeps alone.
And the sea lifts and falls all night, the moon goes on through
    the unattached heavens alone.
The toe of the shoe pivots
in the dust . . .
And the man in the black coat turns, and goes back down
    the hill.

No one knows why he came, or why he turned away, and
   did not climb the hill.

One can feel some mood of the fifth stage in that poem, some
melancholy. I have spoken of the anger I see: flying out toward my
sons, probably an anger passed down from my grandfather to my
father to me, and one aim I felt in raising my sons was not to let
that anger get passed on any farther, at least unconsciously. Part
of that struggle is in a poem called "For My Son Noah, Ten Years
Old."

Night and day arrive, and day after day goes by,
and what is old remains old, and what is young
   remains young, and grows old.
The lumber pile does not grow younger, nor the
   two-by-fours lose their darkness,
but the old tree goes on, the barn stands without help
   so many years;
the advocate of darkness and night is not lost.

The horse steps up, swings on one leg, turns its body,
the chicken flapping claws onto the roost, its wings
   whelping and walloping,
but what is primitive is not to be shot out into the
   night and the dark.
And slowly the kind man comes closer, loses his rage,
   sits down at table.

So I am proud only of those days that pass in
   undivided tenderness,
when you sit drawing, or making books, stapled,
   with messages to the world,
or coloring a man with fire coming out of his hair.
Or we sit at a table, with small tea carefully poured.
So we pass our time together, calm and delighted.

The end of the poem suggests that spontaneity reappears in our relationship with our children when we live in the grief of the return. To hint more at the mood of the fifth stage, I'll tell two stories, one brief and one long. Mulla Nasrudin one day was out walking with his students when a duck flying over shit in his eye. "Mulla," said the students, "this is terrible! We must get some toilet paper!" "Oh, don't bother," Mulla said, "you couldn't catch him now."

The second story is a tale George Docsi, the architect and author of the book *The Power of Limits*, told me about his childhood in Hungary. His story went something like this: When I was a boy I loved dinner. I loved to go into the dining room and sit in front of the big plates, and have the maid come in and serve the soup. One evening I went downstairs, and the dining room was in an uproar. A pogrom had taken place in Russia, and many Jews were fleeing over the border into our town. My grandfather went down to the railway station and brought home Jews whom he found there. I didn't know what was going on, but I could see old men with skull caps in the living room, mothers nursing babies in the corners of the dining room, and I threw a fit. I said, "I want my supper! I want my supper!" One of the maids offered me a piece of bread. I threw it on the floor and screamed, "I want my supper!" My grandfather happened to enter the room at that moment and heard me. He bent down and picked up the piece of bread, kissed it, and gave it to me. And I ate it.

Most fathers in such a scene are liable to get angry—I have done it so often with my children—and shout at the child and say, "Pick it up! Children are starving in Africa!" or some idiocy of that sort. George's grandfather skipped that whole scene and himself bent down, yet the child in no way compelled that. Then the kissing of the bread is very beautiful, I'm not sure why. It doesn't accuse the bread of being wicked, or the child, and the act is spontaneous, decisive, and full of true authority and genuine grief. George Docsi later said, "You know, I think there's a little of my grandfather in me now."

So the person who has eaten his shadow spreads calmness, and shows more grief than anger. If the ancients were right that darkness contains intelligence and nourishment and even information, then the person who has eaten some of his or her shadow is more energetic as well as more intelligent.

It is proper to ask then, "How does one go about eating the shadow or retrieving a projection, practically?"

In daily life one might suggest making the sense of smell, taste, touch, and hearing more acute, making holes in your habits, visiting primitive tribes, playing music, creating frightening figures in clay, playing the drum, being alone for a month, regarding yourself as a genial criminal. A woman might try being a patriarch at odd times of the day, to see how she likes it, but it has to be playful. A man might try being a witch at odd times of the day, and see how it feels, but it has to be done playfully. He might develop a witch laugh and tell fairy stories, as the woman might develop a giant laugh and tell fairy stories.

For the man, when he figures out which woman or women are holding his witch, he can go to that woman, greet her cordially, and say, "I want my witch back. Give it to me." A curious smile will come over her face, and she may hand it back or she may not. If she does the man should excuse himself, turn to the left, facing the wall, and eat it. A woman might go to her mother with a similar request, for mothers often hold a daughter's witch, as a form of power. A woman might go to her father and say, "You have my giant. I want it back." Or she may go to an old teacher or ex-husband (or husband) and say, "You have my negative patriarch. I want him back." Even if the person who carries the witch or giant or dwarf is dead, the encounter is often helpful.

There are many other ways to eat the shadow, or retrieve the projection, or lessen the length of the bag, and we all know dozens of them. I'll mention the use of careful language, by which I mean language that is accurate and has a physical base. Using language consciously seems to be the most fruitful method of retrieving shadow substance scattered out on the world. Energy we have sent out is floating around beyond the psyche; and one way to pull it back into the psyche is by the rope of language. Certain kinds of language are nets, and we need to use the net actively, throwing it out. If we want our witch back we write about her; if we want our spiritual guide back we write about the spiritual guide rather than passively experience the guide in another person. Language contains retrieved shadow substance of all of our ancestors, as Isaac Bashevis Singer or Shakespeare makes clear. If language doesn't seem right at the moment, painting or sculpture may be right, or making images with watercolors. When we paint the witch with conscious intention, we soon find out whose house she's in. So the fifth stage involves activity, imagination, hunting, asking. "Always cry for what you want."

People who are passive toward their projected material contribute to the danger of nuclear war, because every bit of energy that we don't actively engage with language or art is floating somewhere in the air above the United States, and Reagan can use it. He has a big energy sweeper that pulls it in. No one should make you feel guilty for not keeping a journal, or creating art, but such activity helps the whole world. What did Blake say?— "No person who is not an artist can be a Christian." He means that a person who refuses to approach his own life actively, using language, music, sculpture, painting, or drawing is a caterpillar dressed in Christian clothes, not a human being. Blake himself engaged his shadow substance with three disciplines: painting, music, and language. He illuminated his own poems, and set them to music. There was no energy around him that politicians could use to project onto another country. One of the things we need to do as Americans is to work hard individually at eating our shadows, and so make sure that we are not releasing energy which can then be picked up by the politicians, who can use it against Russia, China, or the South American countries.

PART 4

Honoring the Shadow:
An Interview with William Booth

4

Honoring the Shadow:
An Interview with William Booth

Booth: The shadow by definition is that part of ourselves that is hidden from us. How do you answer a person who is not aware of having a shadow and asks you where to look for it?

Bly: I asked that question myself of an experienced Jungian analyst at a public talk, passing on a question asked of me. I said, "Suppose that a woman about thirty-five years old living in a small town in Minnesota knows no psychology. How would that woman begin the process of absorbing her shadow?" His answer was this: unless she meets a teacher who understands the concept of the shadow, she doesn't have a chance. "That's a harsh answer!" I said. "Well," he added, "there might be another way." He observed that our psyche in daily life tries to give us a hint of where our shadow lies by picking out people to hate in an irrational way. Suppose there is a woman in the town who seems to her too loose and too sexually active, and she finds herself thinking of this other woman a lot. In that case, the psyche is suggesting that part of her shadow, at least, lies in the sexual area. She has to notice precisely whom she hates. That is the path of attention. Suppose that she hates the current president of the PTA; and if you ask her, she'll say that the woman is fakey, can't be trusted, is too successful, and so forth. The psyche might be telling her that part of her shadow lies in the power area. She has unused and unrecognized power impulses, which she has put into the bag. Otherwise there wouldn't be such heavily emotional contact with that other person. So, following the path of attention, one notices where the anger goes, and precisely whom we become obsessed with. We become entangled with people who are virtually strangers. That's odd. The metaphor is this: if we maintain eye contact with that person, we can damage him or her by our anger and hatred. If we break off eye contact and look down quickly to the right, we will see our own shadow. Hatred then is very helpful. The old tradition says that if a man loves God he can become holy in twenty years; but if he hates God he can do the same work in two years.

Paying attention to what one likes or hates in literature helps also. I've always been obsessed with certain eighteenth-century men, Pope and Johnson, for example. I grumble about them as neoclassical, haters of feeling, rationalistic sticks, followers of metrical rules, enemies of spontaneity, etc. I finally stopped attacking them, and looked down to the right: it's obvious that I've had in me for years an unused and unrecognized classical side, and I have to readjust my view of my own openness to feeling. It's possible I'm not romantic. Facing that had two effects: first, I wasn't able to sustain my hatred for Samuel Johnson. As a matter of fact, I find his essay on Milton absolutely magnificent. And second, I have to realize that other people see in me the very thing I saw in Johnson, and who is to say they are wrong?

Booth: So we are particularly sensitive to a quality in someone else that we have been burying in ourselves?

Bly: Yes. The peculiarity of our shadow lies in what we are burying. I for example have longed to think of myself as a nice person, that is, responsible, decent, thoughtful, etc. This is one of the major efforts I make. I have been told that I should be a nice person. As far as we know, this is not something the old Celts were told in the time of Cuchulain. They were told that you were to be a daring person, a brave person. You were never to whine; even at the moment of death you were to tell jokes. That would have quite different results. So their shadow probably lay in cowardice and in melancholy. Our shadow tends, because our parents urged unselfishness on us, to lie in being greedy or sneaky, wanting fame without deserving it, being an operator. Were you brought up to be nice?

Booth: Of course. It's still a big problem.

Bly: We bump into that problem in the men's groups. The Widow Douglas wanted Huck Finn to be nice. And after he has floated down the river with the black man, Aunt Sally wants to adopt him and "civilize" him. Huck says, "I can't stand it. I been there before."

Let me give you one more answer to the question, "How do I know I have a shadow?" The other day I was making coffee for Ruth and myself. I put a spoon and a half of ground coffee in her filter and the same in mine. Then something inside me reached back and took another half spoonful for mine. It wasn't me—I didn't do it. I just noticed it happen.

Booth: I once heard a man say about a certain placid young woman that she had no shadow. Is it possible for someone not to have a shadow?

Bly: Have you ever seen anyone walk in the sun and yet the shadow was missing?

Booth: It would have to be a very thin person.

Bly: Terribly thin. Perhaps transparent.

Booth: But transparency could imply either that a person is insubstantial or that he or she has nothing to hide.

Bly: It is said that some old Zen people have done so much work on their shadow that they will do greedy things right in front of you and laugh. By showing the greediness directly, in daylight, somehow they bring it out of the world of shadow and into the world of play. It is said that old Zen people stop dreaming. It is possible that one of the reasons that all of us dream so much is that the dreamer wants to remind us of the amount of shadow that we haven't absorbed. I would think it possible that a sixty-five- or seventy-year-old person could be transparent. But the woman was in her twenties?

Booth: Yes.

Bly: I'd say there's no chance. Such a woman might even say that she doesn't dream, but if you checked her rapid eye movements, you would see that she dreams quite a bit.

Booth: So such a person is not aware of the shadow, but it is there.

Bly: It is inconceivable that at twenty-eight we could have lived out everything. Our shadow includes a whole landscape. Some of our shadow, in the 20th century, obviously hides in the sexual area, for example—in sexual greediness, sexual brutality—and pornography makes that clear. But I believe that there is also a hunter and hermit area of the shadow, containing various primitive impulses that have nothing to do with sexuality—maybe a desire to live in the woods, a desire to kill animals and smear their blood on our faces, a desire to get away from all profane life and live religiously like an Australian aborigine. There is no way we can live all that material. Then there is an abundant landscape where the emotions of hatred, fear, anger, jealousy live. We have a bigger store of those at birth than we are able to live out. Just think how angry and irritable we get if an airline clerk makes a mistake! At least I do. So I have been thinking of the shadow as threefold.

I read an article in *Psychology Today*, and the gist of it is that in China the children are not allowed to speak or act out their negative emotions. If a child expresses anger, the mother will put two fingers to her cheek and say, "Shame!" She will respond similarly to competitiveness or greed. The child, then, is taught politeness toward parents, noncompetitiveness toward brothers and sisters; and if he has anger, he is taught not to express it. Jung said that when the shadow is successfully repressed, the person doing it finds it very difficult to talk to other people about feelings. The people who wrote this article report that in a Chinese family very little discussion of feelings takes place. The child almost never talks with his parents about his or her feelings, never with brothers and sisters; the child sometimes talks about feelings with cousins. Luckily there are many cousins in the Chinese extended family. The shadow of the Chinese, then, would seem to have its foothold in the third area, the area of hatred, fear, anger, and jealousy.

In our culture, as a result of permissive theories of childrearing, kindergarten teachers, or some of them, still think it is good if the child expresses anger, gets the aggression "out of his system"—that's the phrase that is used often. With us, some children are urged to express their anger. So that part of their shadow becomes visible, appears in broad daylight.

Booth: This sounds like an antidote to the problem of stuffing things into the bag.

Bly: The planners intended it as an antidote. Yet the plan has not worked very well. I'm not sure that the expression of the sexual material in the young has worked out very well either. The problem is this: whenever a kindergarten child expresses violent anger and acts it out, it's as if the electrical impulse makes a path in the brain down which the anger can go even more easily next time. But explosive anger is often felt by the ego as a defeat. The ego is in charge of making a social being out of us. If the child's tantrum angers an adult, the child's ego may be damaged by what happens next. When the child brought up permissively becomes forty or fifty years old, he may still be acting out anger in the kindergarten way, as electricity passes along the old grooves in the brain. The person is not strengthened, but in fact is humiliated, by these explosions of anger.

Booth: So the child has to experience freedom of expression, but also experience a strengthening of the ego.

Bly: Well, it's as if there were some kind of game being played here between the ego and the shadow. When permissive educators come in and tell children to express their anger, it's like giving the shadow side fifteen balls and the structure side none. Permissiveness is a misunderstanding of the seriousness of that game. George Leonard, in his book called *The End of Sex*, describes himself as having been enthusiastic about the complete expression of sexuality during the sixties. He now feels that such expression results eventually in some humiliation of the ego, and the psyche as a result loses some of its interest in sexuality; it loses some of its eros.

The culture has a longing for primitive modes of expression as an antidote to repression. Nazi youth groups emphasized a kind of back-to-nature primitivism. Obviously Nazism involved a state insanity, and not all back-to-nature movements involve insanity; most embody health. And yet we can understand through Kurtz's experience in *Heart of Darkness* that the Western longing for the primitive is dangerous to the psyche. The ego becomes unable to hold its own among the primitive impulses and dissolves in mass movements, vanishes like sugar in water.

Booth: I notice that most people who talk about a "personal shadow" or a "national shadow" have trouble keeping the term "shadow" neutral. "Shadow" and "dark side of the self" have negative connotations and associations with evil.

Bly: This tendency to associate the dark side with evil came up very interestingly in some responses to the interview that Keith Thompson and I did in *New Age* a couple of years ago about the wild man. You remember that we discussed a scene in the Grimm brothers' story "Iron John," in which after men bucket out a pond they find a man entirely covered with hair lying at the bottom. As we experienced the responses from men and women who wrote or spoke to us, it became clear that we failed to make one important distinction—the distinction between the wild man and the savage man. We're going to make it in the next interview. Our language includes in its spectrum the tame, obedient man, on one end, and the savage, represented by men who rape women on pool tables, on the other end. There is no place in the psyche for the wild man who is neither. A few men took the image of the wild man as permission for being savage, failing to make any distinction.

When the Los Angeles *Free Press* reprinted that interview, a woman psychoanalyst, German by birth, wrote to the newspaper and said something like this: "There is something we have to make very clear, and that is that this person under the water is a *killer!*" But Iron John throughout the story behaves in a gentle, even courtly way. She took her grasp of what happened in Germany and imposed it upon this particular story. To say it another way, she had no room in her mind in which the concept of the wild man could live; the walls between the rooms had been broken down by the savage man, who occupied the wild man's room as well as his own.

We could distinguish between the wild man and the savage man by looking at several details: the wild man's possession of spontaneity, the presence of the female side in him, and his embodiment of positive male sexuality. None of these implies violence toward or domination of others. I feel that the man under the water resembles a Zen priest more than a so-called primitive who in our view would only grunt. The image of the wild man describes a state of soul that allows shadow material to return slowly in such a way that it doesn't damage the ego. Apparently what we're hearing in "Iron John" is a narrative reminder of old initiation rituals in northern Europe. The older males would teach the younger males how to deal with shadow material in such a way that it doesn't overwhelm the ego or the personality. They taught the encounter more as a kind of play than as a fight.

When the shadow becomes absorbed the human being loses much of his darkness and becomes light and playful in a new way. The unabsorbed shadow can darken the air all around a human being. Pablo Casals is an example of the first type, and Cotton Mather of the second.

Booth: I'm confused by your use of the word "light" in this context—saying that a person who absorbs the shadow becomes not dark, but light and playful. You have sometimes used the word "light" in a negative sense. In your 1971 shadow reading you said that Bertrand Russell had too much light in his personality. You wanted a political leader who was a crow, not a dove or a swallow.

Bly: OK—then I'll withdraw the term "light." Marie Louise von Franz says somewhere that a human being who has done work with the shadow or absorbed the shadow gives a sense of being condensed. Other people willingly give him or her some authority in moral matters. If a teacher has worked with his own shadow, she says that students, no matter how young they are, sense it, and discipline in that room will not be difficult, because the students know that the teacher has his crow with him. Other teachers, she says, who have not worked with their shadow, can talk about discipline all day and never get it. I like the idea that the work a person does on his or her shadow results in a condensation, a thickening or a densening, of the psyche which is immediately apparent, and which results in a feeling of natural authority without the authority being demanded.

Booth: Do you see that quality in any of our political leaders?

Bly: Ronald Reagan has certainly not absorbed his shadow. There is nothing condensed about him at all. We know that he is still projecting his shadow on Russia, which he calls an evil empire. And he insists that desperate farmers in El Salvador are all puppets of Russia. He's drawing on a fund of wise-father-longing which Americans project on him. Winston Churchill did absorb his shadow, and he exercised a natural authority. There was something extremely infantile in him—that's where his shadow lay—but he seems to have faced that and eaten it. Do you see anyone in politics who has a good condensed feeling about him?

Booth: My mind went back to Lincoln. I think he had a

tremendous moral authority that went along with a lack of illusion about himself and his causes. He wasn't sanctimonious.

Bly: Another quality that comes in when a person absorbs his shadow is a certain kind of humor. Lincoln had it. Someone asked Lincoln if he would find him a good government job, and Lincoln said, "I have very little influence in this administration." When a woman he met on a train told him he was one of the ugliest men she'd seen in her entire life, he didn't become offended. "What should I do about that?" he asked the woman. "Well," she said, "you could stay home." Lincoln told that story on himself—he liked her answer.

Booth: You gave a reading in the late sixties that I remember, and you seemed exhilarated then by the evidence of shadow in America—in long hair, rock music, new interest in art, the emergence of good poetry such as Gary Snyder's and Galway Kinnell's. You said, "It's a wonderful movement; we're all returning to the shadow." How does that movement look to you now?

Bly: If we had done any work in truly absorbing the shadow, some shift, however small, would have occurred in the whole American psyche in the direction of an ability to admit our dark side. It's clear that no such change has taken place.

It is said that inside our body there is a vast gap—perhaps thousands of miles across—between the power chakra in the stomach and the heart chakra in the chest. I remember a scene once at Ojai. Some gentle Krishnamurti people asked Joseph Campbell, at one of his lectures, about the spiritual seed brought from India to California in the 1920s by Vivekananda and others. Didn't he think that this seed was already working, and that a new stage in world culture had already begun? Joseph said, "I can't assure you of that. As a matter of fact, it is my opinion that the popular culture never gets above the power chakra." That's a stark and fierce view. It coincides, by the way, with the theme of power over others that one always hears in the Nashville lyrics, and the obsession of popular movies with power—the

James Bond movies—as distinguished from love or spirit. If Campbell is right, mass culture will never teach the absorption of the shadow. If a person is to absorb the shadow, he or she would have to move up to the heart area. Since popular culture did dominate the sixties, I was wrong to imagine that the culture as a whole could move out of the power chakra. Many of us were wrong about that.

Another way to put it is that people under thirty-five cannot teach themselves or others to eat the shadow. The initiation rituals hinted at in "Iron John" imply and suppose old men who teach younger men how to eat the shadow. That teaching did not appear in the sixties, and it's not appearing now. Old men like Reagan, in fact, are teaching younger males how to project their shadow, not how to eat it. Reagan teaches a kind of genial commercial paranoia, so I don't think things look hopeful.

Let's go back again to this game that the ego plays with the unlived material. Baker Roshi, during a little talk one day, remarked that ordinarily in our culture we have only two ideas: either we express or we repress. Either one represses anger or one expresses it. For example, it could be said that Richard Straus is repressing certain negative emotions, whereas punk rock is expressing them. But expressing is not any more admirable then repressing. The Western man or woman lives in a typical pairing of opposites that destroys the soul. Either we defeat Communism or we are defeated by it. Either a man dominates women or he is dominated by them. Joseph Campbell describes the two opposites as two horns; and if we get hooked on either, we die. Baker Roshi remarked that in Zen the student tries to imagine a third possibility. It goes like this. In meditation, he said, one might allow the anger to come in, so that the whole body burns with anger. The anger is not repressed; your whole body *is* anger. One may want to feel that anger for three or four hours. During this time one is neither expressing it nor repressing it. Then, when the meditation ends, one has the choice to express the anger or not. The ego or personality can make the choice later, to express it or not. Moreover, expressing it might not involve the kind of scarifying scene in which you scream at someone and wear tracks in your brain. In fact, the anger might be expressed by some witticism on the phone that would take twenty seconds, but the listener wouldn't forget it for five years. The personality would find an appropriate way to express anger which would support playfulness, give honor to the anger, and yet not contribute to the disintegration of its own organized psyche.

Booth: As usual, what you are saying requires growth. You're not talking about jumping back to childhood and pulling things out of the bag.

Bly: A woman told me a touching story about jumping back. She was a California woman, and had been invited to a women's conference in northern Minnesota, her first. On the opening night, she said, all of us were nervous, and we didn't say much the first time around. The second time around we said more. The third time around each of us said a lot. By the fourth round, which came the next day, much hurt feeling and anger appeared—the dry-eyed were taking care of weeping women lying on the floor. In the fifth round even more came loose, and everyone was honest. It felt at the time like a tremendous victory. But, she said, a few days later I felt drained and defeated, and nothing had really changed.

The women, bravely, allowed rage, humiliation, jealousy, and anger to be *expressed*, but she concluded that expressing shadow material by itself doesn't help. The act is more savage than wild.

The last thing I want to say about the shadow is an idea I've been thinking about more and more: the matter of honoring the shadow material. If we don't live our animal side or our sexual side, that means we don't *honor* those parts. It has been said that the greatest harm the Christian church has done is to make people mistrust instincts, but who taught us to mistrust our anger? How can we honor our anger and still not express it routinely? And if we have anger and do not make proper clothing for it, but make it live in the closet or else let it run around naked screaming at everybody, that means that we are failing to honor our anger.

Booth: I wish you would say more about how one can honor those negative emotions, including anger.

Bly: Three honorings come to mind. First of all, anger can happen when listening to others talk. If someone tells you, say, of some abuse that he or she has suffered, and describes it in a flat voice, one may feel anger, a kind of sympathetic anger. One could capture and honor that anger, and instinctively trust it, allowing it to take shape in words. "I feel some anger listening to this story."

Secondly, Marie Louise suggests that we regard our anger as a person and talk to it. Rather than acting as a conduit for our own anger, and focusing it on another person, one turns one's face and body to the anger itself, and asks: "What do you want from me? What do you want of me?" That is honoring the anger, just as we honor everyone whom we turn to face.

Booth: It seems to me that this would apply to anything in the shadow.

Bly: I think so. We can ask our sexuality: "What do you want from me?" We could ask of our infantilism: "What do you want me to do?"

Thirdly, it's possible that we keep in touch with our anger only enough to make a shady deal with it, not out in the open. We relate to our anger the way Mafia bosses in New Jersey relate to petty mobsters. A guy comes slinking in and the bosses pay him fifty bucks to do a job for them. Then when he comes back they can't even remember that they told him to do anything, and what's worse, if anyone goes to the pen, he's the one. I have, and we may all have, an underground, under-the-table, shady deal going with our anger, so that it does certain things for us. We ourselves look fine socially—we answer questions calmly, we adopt Robert's rules of order—and yet all that time our anger is doing a lot of damage to people around us. I have mentioned that we lose energy whenever these shadow powers are allowed to operate under the table. But we would also have to say that the danger is not only the danger of losing energy; there is the question of the anger itself being angry at us. The anger is angry with us for not honoring it, for treating it shabbily, for getting out of it what we want without ever bringing it in and introducing it to our friends, saying, "This is my friend Anger here. He's a lowly-paid assistant of mine."

Booth: I try to keep him out of sight, but he does some damage to my friends once in a while.

Bly: The question is, what is the anger doing to you? When does he really plan to fix you? Now, what haven't we said about the shadow?

Booth: We've talked little about the relationship between shadow and evil. It is clear that the shadow is not to be identified with evil, but how does evil fit in?

Bly: Well, let's try to make a distinction. The shadow energies seem to be a part of the human psyche, a part of its 360-degree nature, and the shadow energies become destructive only when they are ignored. The shadow energies remain a part of or belong to the human community. But our ancestors, some of them, had a sense that evil is something quite different. It comes from beyond the human community; it flows in from an archaic principle that still exists in the universe—many Gnostics believed that—or from the dead, who have passed out of the human community. And from that point of view evil can be dealt with or recognized, but not absorbed. We know it's dangerous to imagine that we could have friendly relationships with all forms of destructive energy. Such humanistic confidence is too optimistic. There may be powers in the universe outside the human community and hostile to the human community. But our conversation has been about shadow primarily.

Booth: We come back then to the idea that the shadow is what is hidden from us, and it is not something destructive in its very essence. I recall your poem "The Moon," written some years ago, that carries this sense of the shadow.

Bly: It goes like this.

> After writing poems all day,
> I went off to see the moon on the piney hill.
> Far in the woods I sit down against a pine.
> The moon has her porches turned to face the light,
> but the deep part of her house is in darkness.

PART 5

Wallace Stevens and Dr. Jekyll

5

Wallace Stevens and Dr. Jekyll

The literature of the American earth is many thousands of years old, and its rhythms are still rising from the serpents buried in Ohio, from the shells the Yakuts ate of and threw to the side. The literature of the American nation is only two hundred years old. How much of the darkness from under the earth has risen into poems and stories in that time?

All literature, both of the primitive and the modern peoples, can be thought of as creations by the "dark side" to enable it to rise up from earth and join the sunlit consciousness again. Many ancient religions, especially those of the matriarchies, evidently moved so as to bring the dark side up into the personality slowly and steadily. The movement started early in the person's life and, in the Mysteries at least, lasted for twenty to thirty years. Christianity, as many observers have noticed, has acted historically to polarize the "dark personality" and the "light personality." Christian ethics usually involves the suppression of the dark one. As the consequences of this suppression become more severe, century after century, we reach at last the state in which the psyche is split, and the two sides cannot find each other. We have "The Strange Story of Dr. Jekyll and Mr. Hyde." The dominant personality in the West tends to be idealistic, compassionate, civilized, orderly, as Dr. Jekyll's, who is so caring with his patients; the shadow side is deformed, it moves fast, "like a monkey," is younger than the major personality, has vast sources of energy near it, and no morality at all. It "feels" rage from centuries of suppression.

How did the two persons get separated? Evidently we spend the first twenty or twenty-five years of life deciding what should be pushed down into the shadow self, and the next forty years trying to get in touch with that material again. Cultures vary a lot in what they urge their members to exile. In general we can say that "the shadow" represents all that is instinctive in us. Whatever has a tail and lots of hair is in the shadow. People in secular and Puritanical cultures tend to push sexual desire into the shape under our feet, and also fear of death; usually much ecstasy goes with them. Old cave impulses go there, longings to eat the whole world—if we put enough down there, the part left on top of the earth looks quite respectable.

Conrad is a great master of shadow literature; *The Secret Sharer* describes the healing of the same split that Stevenson could not heal. Conrad suspects that at times the shadow will not rejoin the consciousness unless the person has a serious task, which he accepts, such as captaining a ship. *Heart of Darkness* describes a failure in the same effort. Conrad noticed that the European solved his shadow problem less often after the invasion of Africa. The European now has a financial interest in the suppression of the shadow. Kurtz's history suggests that for a white man to recover his shadow at the same time he is exploiting blacks is a task beyond the power of the human being.

This speculation sends reverberations through American fiction also, both North and South. Mark Twain makes a similar point in *Huckleberry Finn*, brilliantly, joyously. Sometimes in the United States the "decent man" is hidden in the shadow, along with a lot of other stuff, and, as Huckleberry Finn finds out, the "decent man" will rejoin you only if you refuse to sell Jim.

Most of our literature describes efforts the shadow makes to rise, and efforts that fail. Ahab fails; it isn't clear why; he has a strong connection with the "old ethic" through the rhetoric of the Hebrew prophets. Dimmesdale's shadow fails. Apparently his fear of women blocks his own shadow from rising. I prefer to use the term "shadow," rather than "evil," in talking of literature, because "evil" permanently places the energy out there, as a part of some powerful being other than ourselves. "Shadow" is clumsy, but it makes it clear that these energies are inside of us.

Alexandra David-Neel tells a disturbing story. When she was studying with some Tibetan teachers early in this century, they suggested she try to get a clearer experience of her life-energy or libido. They suggested that she put it outside herself, where she could see it more clearly, and not into objects, but into a thought-form, a figure she herself would visualize and which would not exist outside of her head. She decided not to choose a typical Tibetan visualization—some energetic dancing figure, with necklaces of skulls, and flames coming out of the hairs on his chest—on the grounds that she herself might consider it to be a simple transfer from a Tibetan unconscious. She decided instead to visualize an English monk of the Middle Ages. After a few weeks of visualization, which she did among some other duties, she noticed one day, while walking outside the monastery on the road, an English monk dressed in gray who approached and passed her. After several such meetings, he began to greet her when they met, and she could see his eyes. He would disappear if she "unthought" him. Soon, however, she noticed that he was growing bolder; he appeared to be drawing energy from her without her will, and to be taking on a life of his own. She became frightened then. Eventually she went to her Tibetan teacher, who taught her how to perform a rather long ritual to get rid of the monk. A man or woman who talks of evil in *Moby Dick* is the kind of person who would believe that monk was real.

The group of American poets born from 1875 to 1890, namely Wallace Stevens, Frost, Eliot, Williams, Marianne Moore, Pound, and Jeffers, are all shadow poets. They are not only shadow poets, but they did much shadow work. Most shadow work appeared in novel form in the last century; in this century it has tended to appear in poetry. Wallace Stevens is usually not thought of as a shadow writer, so we can take him; and his work will have to stand for the others in that marvelous group.

It is interesting to compare Wallace Stevens's background with Kenneth Rexroth's, as it appears in Rexroth's autobiography. The Rexroths tended to live out their shadow. Stevens's family, upper middle-class German Americans, appear to be successful repressors of the dark side. How the shadow returns in a complicated man like Wallace Stevens I don't know; I don't understand the return of the shadow at all well, and everything I say here is speculation. But it seems the shadow energies need special channels in order to return. Eliot's sharp griefs, coming first in his marriage, and followed then by his wife's insanity, are linked with the rising of much shadow energy in him, but none of that violent anguish appears in Stevens. In Stevens shadow material rises in perfect serenity, associated with the awakening of the senses, especially of hearing and smell. Our senses do form a natural bridge to our animal past, and so to the shadow. The senses of smell, shades of light and dark, the awareness of color and sound, so alive in the primitive man, for whom they can mean life or death, are still alive in us, but numbed. They are numbed by safety, and by years inside schoolrooms. Wallace Stevens, it seems, when he was working in insurance early on, would try to end the day at some New England town that had a museum. He would then spend a couple of hours looking at pictures. This is a practical way of reawakening the senses, as walks are. Both reawaken more of the senses than reading does.

> Among twenty snowy mountains,
> The only moving thing
> Was the eye of the blackbird.

It is said that eyes in the West receive a disproportionate amount of psychic energy; all the other senses have become weakened to the degree that reading has laid emphasis on sight. The old harmony between the five senses has been destroyed. Stevens is careful of hearing:

I do not know which to prefer,
The beauty of inflections
Or the beauty of innuendoes,
The blackbird whistling
Or just after.

. . .

It was evening all afternoon.
It was snowing
And it was going to snow.
The blackbird sat
In the cedar-limbs.

The last poem has the most marvelous and alert sense for changes of light, the deepening darkness, sensed with the body, as snow is about to fall. He pays more attention than most men to uniting the senses of color and smell:

The night is of the color
Of a woman's arm:
Night, the female,
Obscure,
Fragrant and supple,
Conceals herself.
A pool shines,
Like a bracelet
Shaken in a dance.

He works to join the eyes to the sense of touch:

The light is like a spider. . . .
The webs of your eyes
Are fastened
To the flesh and bones of you
As to rafters or grass.

> There are filaments of your eyes
> On the surface of the water
> And in the edges of the snow.

He works to become aware of weather, and its mergings with
emotion:

> Passions of rain, or moods in falling snow;
> Grievings in loneliness, or unsubdued
> Elations when the forest blooms; gusty
> Emotions on wet roads on autumn nights;

He begins to see how, if the senses are sharpened by labor, you
begin to merge with the creatures and objects around you:

> I am what is around me.

> Women understand this.
> One is not duchess
> A hundred yards from a carriage.

Curious and mysterious substances rise in the poems when he
starts to glide out on the rays of his senses:

> He rode over Connecticut
> In a glass coach.
> Once, a fear pierced him,
> In that he mistook
> The shadow of his equipage
> For blackbirds.

That describes a pure shadow instant, in which shadow mate-
rial shoots up into the conscious mind. Often, when the shadow
shoots up into consciousness for a split second, it brings with it
the knowledge that we will die. Oddly, concentration on ants
sometimes carries that information to the consciousness:

I measure myself
Against a tall tree.
I find that I am much taller,
For I reach right up to the sun,
With my eye;
And I reach to the shore of the sea
With my ear.
Nevertheless, I dislike
The way the ants crawl
In and out of my shadow.

I would guess it would be difficult for readers who read Stevens
in translation to understand the shadow energy moving so ele-
gantly through the senses, because the extraordinary richness of
his sensual intelligence appears as delicate auras surrounding the
words in English, as a perfume surrounds each sort of metal and
each tree. Readers brought up in English whose sense of language
has been coarsened by too much newspaper reading probably
don't feel the complicated aura around Stevens's words either.

By this light the salty fishes
Arch in the sea like tree-branches,
Going in many directions
Up and down.

Senses intersect in those phrases. It is the opposite of academic
poetry or philosophic diction. Stevens notices that:

It is better that, as scholars,
They should think hard in the dark cuffs
Of voluminous cloaks . . .

Basho said, listening in his garden to a temple bell:
The temple bell stops—
but the sound keeps coming
out of the flowers.

Basho worked both as a Buddhist meditator and as a haiku poet in awakening the senses:

> The sea grows dark.
> The voices of the wild ducks
> turn white.

American haiku poets don't grasp the idea that the shadow has to have risen up and invaded the haiku poem, otherwise it is not a haiku. The least important thing about it is its seventeen syllables or the nature scene.

The "Harmonium" that Stevens talks of, and wanted, in vain, to use as a title for his *Collected Poems*, refers to this union of all the five senses, and perhaps of eight or nine more that only Australian hunters or Basho could identify. The serenity that gives music to Stevens's lines is a mark of the presence of that ancient union of the senses.

It was amazing to me recently to find out that one of his main helpers in this effort was William James. We ordinarily think of the senses and thought as opposites, so we assume that if one wants to reawaken the senses, one must stop thinking. When I first read *Harmonium* I was surprised to see that the thinking is expressed through odor and sound images, and the sense images become more intense through the thinking going on. What I didn't know is that the thinking is of the sort recommended by William James. Margaret Peterson set all that out in a spirited essay printed in *Southern Review*'s Stevens issue, Summer 1971. It turns out that some of the most enigmatic and vivid poems in *Harmonium* are rephrasings of paragraphs by James. How unpredictable it all is!

William James warned his students that a certain kind of mind-set was approaching the West—it could hardly be called a way of thought—in which no physical details are noticed. Fingernails are not noticed, trees in the plural are mentioned, but no particular tree is ever loved, nor where it stands; the hair in the ear is not noticed. We now see this mind-set spread all over freshman English papers, which American students can now write quickly, on utterly generalized subjects; the nouns are usually plurals, and the feelings are all ones it would be nice to have. The same mind-set turns up on the Watergate tapes, and working now with more elaborate generalizations, in graduate seminars in English, in which all the details in Yeats's poems turn out to be archetypes or Irish Renaissance themes. It is the *lingua franca*, replacing Latin. The mind-set could be described as the ability to talk of Africa without visualizing the hair in a baboon's ear, or even a baboon. Instead the mind-set reports "wild animals." Since the immense range of color belongs to physical detail—the thatness—of the universe, it is the inability to see color. People with this mind-set have minds that resemble white nightgowns. For people with this mind-set, there's not much difference between 3 and 742; the count of something is a detail. In fact the number they are most interested in, as James noted, is one. That's a number without physical detail. As I read Peterson's essay, I was amazed to see "Metaphors of a Magnifico," which I had always loved as a zany poem of high spirits, become a serious process poem. The poem describes how to begin to free yourself from this mind-set; how to avoid being murdered by it. (So Ph.D.'s on *Harmonium* are especially funny.) He begins:

> Twenty men crossing a bridge,
> Into a village,
> Are twenty men crossing twenty bridges,
> Into twenty villages,
> Or one man
> Crossing a single bridge into a village.

He knows he is beginning by singing the sad little song hummed by Ph.D. candidates and politicians and experts in government planning: "One thing equals another thing."

> This is old song
> That will not declare itself . . .

Then he says what to do. Stop juggling ideas. Go to this place with your body, bring the senses forward, sound first, then sight, then smell if possible. Ask your imagination to bring you the sound:

> The boots of the men clump
> On the boards of the bridge.
> The first white wall of the village
> Rises through fruit-trees.
> Of what was it I was thinking?
> So the meaning escapes.
>
> The first white wall of the village . . .
> The fruit-trees . . .

How strange! It is a Purgatory poem, laying out a road, a sort of guru poem. How beautiful!

William James observed the approaching mind-set and associated out from it sideways. He noticed the mind-set resembled the upper class of Boston. They too disliked the sordid details—the hair in the ear of religion, the smells of the Irish entryway—and preferred the religion of the One. Naturally, they became Unitarians. If the "cultured people" move into this mind-set, a curious thing happens: the upper (spiritual) half of life and the lower (sensual) half of life begin to part company. One part ascends; the other part, no longer connected to the high, sinks. The gaps between grow wider and wider. The educated class has the Pure One, the working class people are left with nothing but the crude physical details of their lives—the husband's old pipe and the spit knocked out of it, the washing tub, the water and slush from the children's boots on the entry floor, the corns on the feet, the mess of dishes in the sink, the secular love-making in the cold room. These physical details are now, in the twentieth century, not only unpenetrated by religion, but they somehow prove to the unconscious that "religion is a nullity." James emphasized that perception, and Stevens grieved over the insight all his life. For the working class there's nothing left but the Emperor of Ice Cream. The middle class is now the working class, and so the majority of people in the West are worse off than they were in the Middle Ages.

James also noticed that the presence of this mind-set in India explains why certain Vedanta philosophies are so boring. An Indian meditation teacher, working with Ananda Marga, told me recently that before he did any meditation at all himself, and while he was working as an engineer in a compressor factory in India, he would at night visit the meeting of whatever holy man was in town. After the talk, he would ask the man, from the audience: What is the relation of your path to the poor in India? Usually—I think he said invariably—ten or twelve times in a row—two husky-looking men would come back and escort him out of the hall. Stevens would have understood that. For most holy men in India, the poor are the hair in the ear of India. They prefer the One, who has no hair.

James made sure his students understood a third sideways association, namely, the link of the mind-set to the German idealists. They were represented in England by Bradley and in the United States by Josiah Royce and the Anglo-Hegelians—horrible types, specialists in the One, builders of middle-class castles, and upper-class Usher houses, writers of boring Commencement speeches, creepy otherworldly types, worse than Pope Paul, academics who resembled gray jars, and who would ruin a whole state like Tennessee if put into it; people totally unable to merge into the place where they live—they could live in a valley for years and never become the valley. Antonio Machado, who did all his academic work in philosophy, describes them also:

> Everywhere I've gone I've seen
> excursions of sadness,
> angry and melancholy
> drunkards with black shadows,
>
> and academics in offstage clothes
> who watch, say nothing, and think
> they know, because they do not drink wine
> in the ordinary bars.

> Evil men who walk around
> polluting the earth . . .

Machado also remarked:

> Mankind owns four things
> that are no good at sea:
> rudder, anchor, oars,
> and the fear of going down.

If we think of the idealists in terms of Jung's speculations about the shadow, it's clear the idealist is a man or woman who does not want to go down. They plan to go to the grave with the shadow still repressed. The idealists are shadow-haters. They all end as does Dr. Jekyll, with a monkey-like Mr. Hyde scurrying among back buildings elsewhere in the city.

By exclusive interest in "the truth," they exile the shadow, or keep it exiled. . . . When Stevens takes his stand against all that, he takes a stand against perfect Paradises, against abstract churches, against the statistical mentality, against too easy transcendentalizing, too easy ignoring of the tragic:

> The imperfect is our paradise.
> Note that, in this bitterness, delight,
> Since the imperfect is so hot in us,
> Lies in flawed words and stubborn sounds.

Stevens did not make Dimmesdale's mistake. He invited the feminine in; Florida, the moon, convolvulus and coral, glade-boats, sombreros, the soles of feet and grape leaves, cabins in Carolina, and so much sound!

Only the shadow understands the ecstasy of sound. You know the shadow has found a way for part of it to return when you hear the joyful and primitive music of Vincentine, as energetic as Mozart, as insistent as Australian drums:

Yes: you came walking,
Vincentine.
Yes: you came talking.

And what I knew you felt
Came then.
Monotonous earth I saw become
Illimitable spheres of you,
And that white animal, so lean,
Turned Vincentine,
Turned heavenly Vincentine,
And that white animal, so lean,
Turned heavenly, heavenly Vincentine.

So Stevens learned how to go home. He learned that the idealist-Christian-Hebraic insistence that there is one truth is all that is needed to block the shadow from rising forever, for a human being, with his frail psychic processes, so easily altered or ground to a stop. He wrote the clear and sweet poem, "On The Way Home":

It was when I said,
"There is no such thing as the truth,"
That the grapes seemed fatter.
The fox ran out of his hole.

You . . . You said,
"There are many truths,
But they are not parts of a truth."
Then the tree, at night, began to change,

Smoking through green and smoking blue.
We were two figures in a wood.
We said we stood alone.

It was when I said,
"Words are not forms of a single word.

In the sum of the parts, there are only the parts.
The world must be measured by eye";

It was when you said,
"The idols have seen lots of poverty,
Snakes and gold and lice,
But not the truth";

It was at that time, that the silence was largest
And longest, the night was roundest,
The fragrance of the autumn warmest,
Closest and strongest.

After writing such a masterpiece as *Harmonium*, guided by the secret knowledge James offered him in his books, and walking the path—he knew he was walking it—why then is there no more to the story?

Sometimes we look to the end of the tale
where there should be marriage feasts,
and find only, as it were,
black marigolds and a silence.

Critics usually accept the world the poet creates. If he says east is north, they say: Why didn't I think of that before! So Stevens's critics on the whole see constant development in his work, in a chosen direction. But it's not so. The late poems are as weak as is possible for a genius to write; what is worse, most of them have the white nightgown mentality.

There are some good poems, but somehow there are no further marriages in his work. Yeats's work picked up more and more detail as it went on, the sensual shadow began to rise, the instinctual energy throws off its own clown clothes and fills more and more of the consciousness.

Why that did not happen to Stevens I don't know for sure, but I think we have to look to his life for an explanation. Boehme has a note before one of his books, in which he asks the reader not to go farther and read the book unless he is willing to make practical changes as a result of the reading. Otherwise, Boehme says, reading the book will be bad for him, dangerous. We have the sense that Wallace Stevens's relation to the shadow followed a pattern that has since become familiar among American artists: he brings the shadow into his art, but makes no changes in the way he lives. The European artists—at least Yeats, Tolstoy, Gauguin, Van Gogh, Rilke—seem to understand better that the shadow has to be lived too, as well as accepted in the work of art. The implication of all their art is that each time a man or woman succeeds in making a line so rich and alive with the senses, as full of darkness as:

quail
Whistle about us their spontaneous cries

he must from then on live differently. A change in his life has to come as a response to the change in his language. Rilke's work moves on, shifting to deeper and deeper marriages, over wider and wider arcs, and we notice that he was always ready to change his way of living at a moment's notice if the art told him to. He looked one day at a statue for a long time, an old statue centered around ecstatic Apollonianism, and saw that the shape was alive not only in the head parts, but in every square inch of the body, throughout the chest and stomach, all of which dived down toward the genitals: every inch is looking at you, he said. Out of that he drew the conclusion that by tomorrow morning he would have to make some changes in the way he lived. I recall teachers at college laughing at Yeats for a remark he made in his journal during his twenties, something like: It seems to me my rhythms are becoming slack; I think I had better sleep on a board for a while. But that says the same thing as Rilke's poem.

Wallace Stevens was not willing to change his way of life, despite all the gifts he received, and all the advice he read in his own poems. He kept the house fanatically neat, evidently slept in a separate bedroom for thirty or forty years, made his living through the statistical mentality, and kept his business life and poetry life separate—all of which amounted to keeping his dominant personality and his shadow personality separate in his daily life. That was so much true that when he took a literary visitor to his club to eat, it seems Stevens entered and conversed there as a businessman, and warned visitors against eccentric behavior. In 1935, during Mussolini's attack on Ethiopia, when Stevens was 56, he wrote in a letter to Ronald Latimer:

> The Italians have as much right to take Ethiopia from the coons as the coons had to take it from the boa-constrictors.

This sentence was intended to be playful, in part at least, and it does not represent a crime that has to be laid to him. And yet it is a sentence that everyone who loves Stevens's poems has to face sooner or later. It seems to indicate that he was not living his shadow very intensely. He had urged the shadow energies to enter *Harmonium*, but at the point where they might have disturbed the even tenor of his life, or the opinions appropriate to it, he shut the door.

I realize that making serious comment on a group of poems by mentioning details of the author's life violates every canon of New Criticism, canons still very much alive. But surely we must see now that this critical insistence on examining only the work is another example of shadow-hatred and shadow-ignoring. It is an idealist position. William James's and Stevens's warning on the mind-set were rejected, and by the 1940s the idealist position in literature was established, and all of us who began to write in the '40s and '50s felt that fact keenly. The critic's assumption was that the author's life had no bearing whatever on the poem. Eliot helped to bring that attitude about, yet I heard him complain in a hockey stadium in St. Paul around 1957 that one of his poems had recently appeared in an anthology holding eight long poems, and that nothing whatever was said about the authors of the poems—their nationality was not given, nor the century in which they had lived. "They were all dead except me, and opening the book made me feel dead too." The mentality of the anthologist was exactly what Stevens called the mentality of the white nightgown. In any case, by 1950 the idealist position had found a good home in literary criticism, and none of us writing then got much help from it on how to bring our own shadows—or the national shadow—into our poems.

Wallace Stevens's statement at the club—don't talk too much about poetry, or too wildly—is somehow the opposite of Tolstoy, who, when he got ready in his old age to free his serfs, found to his amazement that his wife and two of his daughters were ready for no such thing, but considered them part of the property and dowry, and that was an end of it. He left the house in a blizzard with his youngest daughter, Alexandra, and died in a railway station shortly after. He was willing to change his way of life that late!

That story is probably a bad example, because it implies that changing your way of life involves sensational events, catastrophes, turmoil, leaving wife and children, leaving husband and children, slamming the door in the Ibsen manner. The contrary seems to be true. Enormous changes—divorce, throwing away children, abandoning responsibilities, look to be clear ways to join your shadow again, but oddly that doesn't happen most of the time. When a person divorces, he or she usually sets up a similar life with a different person. All the verbal storms of confessional poetry that the poets and readers have gone through in the last years did not achieve anything for the poet— the poet's shadow is still miles away after the confessional book is written. As Plath's and Sexton's and Berryman's lives made clear, nothing has happened at all, and the death energy is still waiting to pounce on the unintegrated soul.

What is meant by Rilke's "You must change your life" is evidently something more subtle. I don't understand it at all myself, so I can only speculate. Conrad evidently made use of the information the shadow gave him by ceasing to be a ship's captain on the Congo, and so a low-level exploiter of Africa.

Rilke, when he realized what his work was telling him, interrupted his writing of poetry, and spent months watching animals in the zoo, and blind men on the streets, and years alone. He began to ask less from the world, not more. The Taoists would probably say that changing your way of life means giving up having an effect upon the world. It involves "wu-wei," not playing any role. Wu-wei is also translated as doing nothing. Wang Wei said once:

In the old days the serious man was not an important person.
He thought making decisions was too complicated for him.
He took whatever small job came along.
Essentially, he did nothing, like these walnut trees.

His friend P'ei Ti answered this way:

I soon found doing nothing was a great joy to me.
You see, here I am, keeping my ancient promise!
Let's spend today just strolling around these walnut trees.
The two of us will nourish the ecstasies Chuang Tzu loved.

A man has an effect on "the world" mainly through institutions. So we could say that in the second half of life a man should sever his link with institutions. I think the problem is more complicated for women, but I don't understand it. Conceivably for women the change might involve accepting more responsibility for affecting the world.

In any case severing ties with institutions is not a habit in the United States, where a man ordinarily becomes more deeply embedded in the institution, whether it be an insurance company or a university, during his forties and fifties than he ever was earlier. John Barth is a contemporary example of the American artist who tries to bring the shadow into his work, but refuses to live it. His work cannot help but follow the same path as Stevens's—it is an ascent into vacuity, intellectualist complexity, a criticism of dry reason from inside the palace of dry reason.

If the shadow's gifts are not acted upon, it evidently retreats

and returns to the earth. It gives the writer or person ten or fif-
teen years to change his life, in response to the amazing visions
the shadow has brought him—that change may involve only a
deepening of the interior marriage of male and female within
the man or woman—but if that does not happen, the shadow
goes back down, abandoning him, and the last state of that man
is evidently worse than the first. Rilke talks of the shadow
retreating in this poem:

> Already the ripening barberries are red,
> and the old asters hardly breathe in their beds.
> The man who is not rich now as summer goes
> will wait and wait and never be himself.
>
> The man who cannot quietly close his eyes
> certain that there is vision after vision
> inside, simply waiting until nighttime
> to rise all around him in the darkness—
> he is an old man, it's all over for him.
>
> Nothing else will come; no more days will open;
> and everything that does happen will cheat him—
> even you, my God. And you are like a stone
> that draws him daily deeper into the depths.